CANCER COOKBOOK

Delicious and Nutritious Recipes for Cancer Patients and Survivors"

Bonus Inside

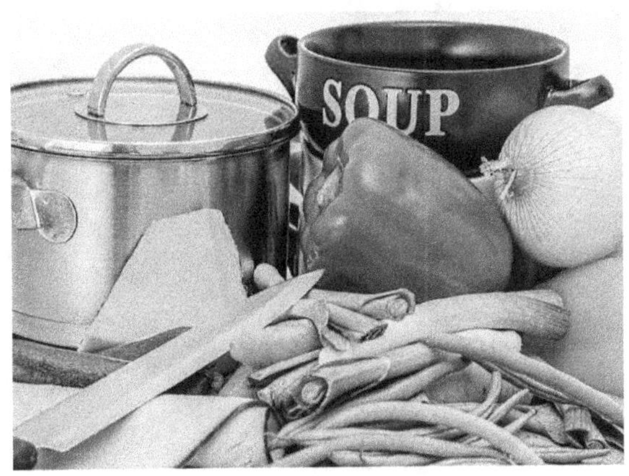

By Laurie C. Spicer

Books by this author:

https://tinyurl.com/448ftvya

https://tinyurl.com/4ak89n48

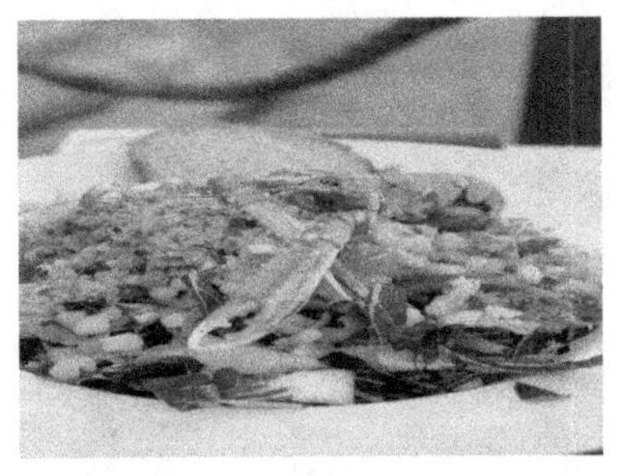

Table of contents

Introduction

Chapter 1 Cancer-fighting breakfast
Anti-Cancer Breakfast Smoothie Recipe
Oatmeal with Superfoods
Avocado Toast with Greens
Eggs with Veggies and Whole Wheat Toast

Chapter 2: Appetizers and Snacks
Guacamole with Fresh Veggies
Cancer-Friendly Hummus Recipe.
Roasted Chickpeas with Spices

Veggie Chips and Salsa
Energy Bites with Nuts and Dried Fruit

Chapter 3: Salads and Dressings
Greek Salad with Grilled Chicken
Rainbow Salad with Quinoa
Spinach Salad with Berries and Nuts
Caesar Salad with Whole Grain Croutons
Balsamic Vinaigrette Dressing
Lemon-Herb Dressing

Chapter 4: Soups and Stews
Vegetable Soup with Lentils
Chicken Noodle Soup with Veggies
Tomato Soup with Whole Grain Crackers
Beef Stew with Root Vegetables
Lentil Stew with Spinach

Chapter 5: Main Dishes
Grilled Salmon with Brown Rice and Steamed Veggies
Whole Wheat Pasta with Tomato Sauce and Grilled Chicken
Stir-Fry with Tofu and Mixed Veggies

Turkey Chili with Beans and Whole Grain Bread
Baked Sweet Potato with Black Beans and Salsa

Chapter 6: Desserts
Fruit Salad with Yogurt and Granola
Chocolate Avocado Pudding
Banana-Oat Cookies with Raisins
Berry Crisp with Whole Grain Topping
Pumpkin Pie with Whole Wheat Crust

Chapter 7 Bonus/ Conclusion
Tips for Meal Planning and Preparation:
Resources for Cancer Patients and Caregivers:

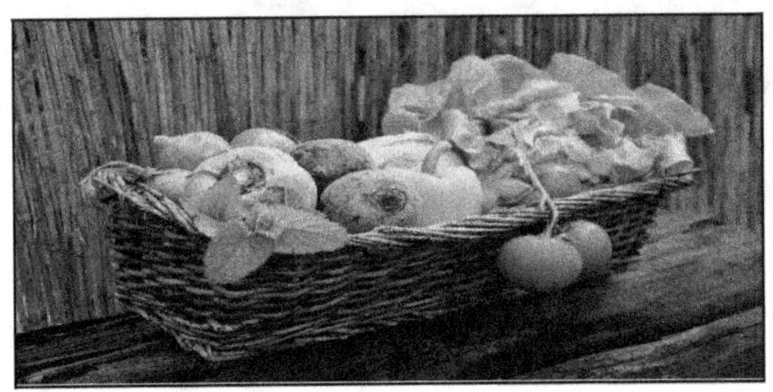

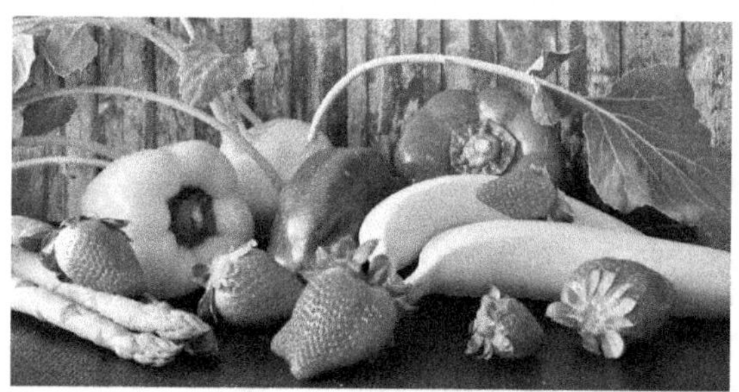

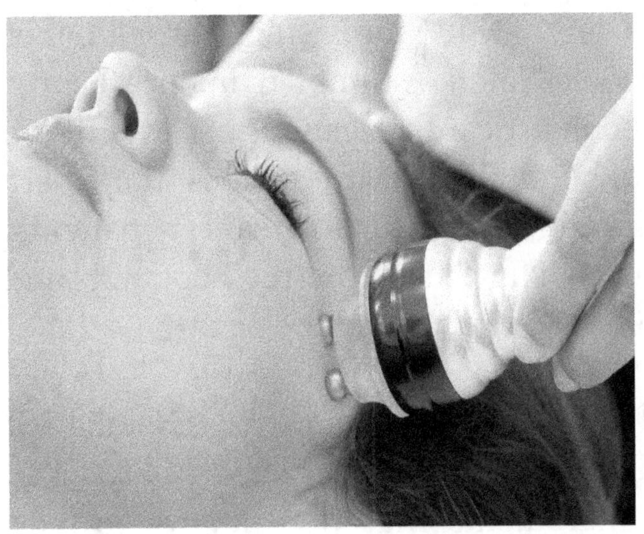

Introduction

Natalia had just received the news that nobody ever wants to hear: she had cancer. The news hit her hard, and she found herself struggling to come to terms with what was happening. She knew that she had a tough road ahead of her, but she was determined to fight.

One day, while browsing through her Facebook Natalia stumbled upon a cancer cookbook article that caught her eye. It was a cookbook filled with recipes that were specifically designed for cancer patients. Intrigued, she clicked on the book link and started reading through the pages.

As she read through the recipes, Natalia felt a sense of hope. Each recipe was packed with ingredients that were known to have cancer-fighting properties. She knew that she had found something special, something that could help her in her battle against cancer.

Natalia began cooking meals from the cookbook every day. She found that the recipes were not only healthy but also delicious. She experimented with different ingredients and flavors, creating new dishes that she would never have thought of before.

As she continued to cook from the cookbook, Natalia noticed that her energy levels were improving. She was no longer feeling as tired and fatigued as she had been before. She also noticed that her overall health was improving, and she was able to manage the side effects of her cancer treatments much better than before.

Natalia's doctors were amazed by her progress. They had never seen a patient who was able to manage cancer so well. So they were forced to asked her what she was doing differently, and she told them about the cookbook. They were so impressed that they began recommending the cookbook to other cancer patients.

Natalia's journey with cancer was not an easy one, but she was grateful for the cookbook that had helped her along the way.

It had given her a sense of hope, and it had shown her that there was something that she could do to fight back against her illness. She continued to cook from the cookbook long after her cancer went into remission, and it remained a constant source of inspiration and strength for her.

After the review of Natalia from the cookbook which happens to be this cookbook, I was determined to put that same cookbook here for anyone who wants to eliminate his or her cancer illness. If you have cancer or know anyone who has cancer, then recommending or getting a copy of this cookbook for them, will be the best form of love and care you could offer them.

Welcome to the Cancer Cookbook, a guide to nourishing your body and soul during one of life's most challenging experiences. This cookbook is designed to provide cancer patients, survivors, and their loved ones with delicious, nutritious recipes that are easy to prepare and enjoyable to eat.

The treatment of cancer can take a toll on the body, affecting appetite, taste, and digestion. Eating well is essential to maintain strength, promote healing, and improve overall quality of life. The Cancer Cookbook is here to help, offering a wide variety of recipes that are tailored to the needs and preferences of cancer patients.

Our recipes are based on the latest research and recommendations from cancer experts, emphasizing whole, nutrient-dense foods that can support the body's natural healing processes. We also recognize that food is more than just fuel; it's a source of comfort, joy, and connection. That's why our recipes are designed to be flavorful, satisfying, and easy to share with family and friends.

Are you looking for a quick snack?, a nourishing meal?, or a special treat to celebrate a milestone?, then Cancer Cookbook has you covered. We hope that these recipes will not only nourish your body, but also provide a sense of comfort and support during this challenging time.

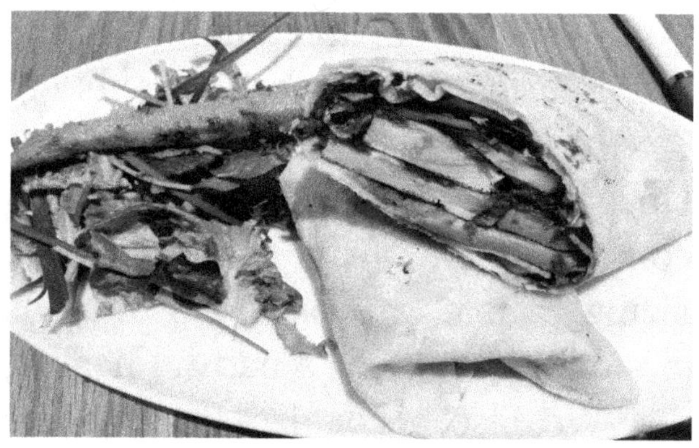

Chapter 1 Cancer-fighting breakfast

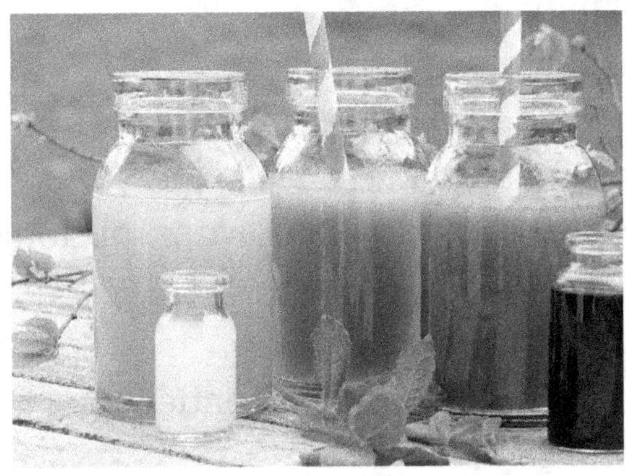

Anti-Cancer Breakfast Smoothie Recipe

Prep time: 5 minutes

Ingredients:

1 cup unsweetened almond milk
1/2 cup frozen mixed berries
1/2 banana
1/2 cup fresh spinach
1 tbsp ground flaxseed
1 tbsp chia seeds
1 scoop vanilla protein powder (optional)
Instructions:

Add all ingredients to a blender.
Blend until smooth.
Pour into a glass and enjoy!
Calories: approximately 300 calories per serving (may vary depending on the brand and type of protein powder used)

Note: This recipe can be easily customized to your liking. You can use different types of milk, berries, or greens to switch up the flavor. You can also add other ingredients like nut butter, coconut oil, or spices like cinnamon or ginger for added health benefits.

Oatmeal with Superfoods

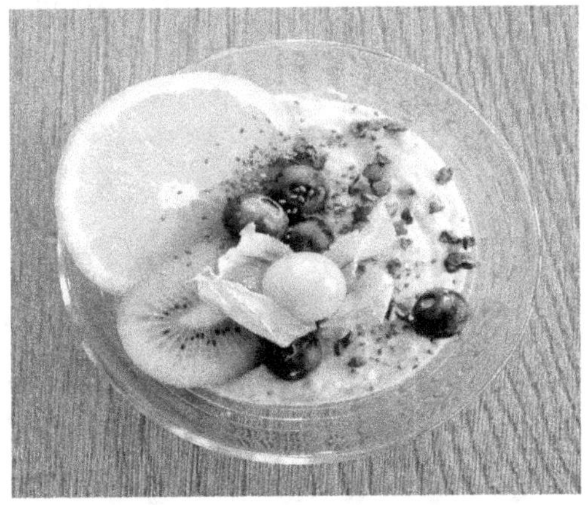

Prep time: 10 minutes

Ingredients:

1/2 cup rolled oats

1 cup unsweetened almond milk (or any milk of your choice)
1/2 teaspoon cinnamon
1/2 teaspoon vanilla extract
1 tablespoon chia seeds
1 tablespoon hemp hearts
1 tablespoon ground flaxseed
1/2 cup mixed berries (fresh or frozen)
1 tablespoon honey or maple syrup (optional)

Instructions:

In a small saucepan, combine the oats, almond milk, cinnamon, and vanilla extract. Bring to a boil over medium-high heat, then reduce the heat to low and simmer for 5-7 minutes, stirring occasionally, until the oatmeal is creamy and thick.
Stir in the chia seeds, hemp hearts, and ground flaxseed.
Serve the oatmeal in a bowl and top with mixed berries and a drizzle of honey or maple syrup, if desired.

Calories: Approximately 400 calories, depending on the type and amount of milk used and the sweetener added.

This recipe is a great source of fiber, protein, healthy fats, and antioxidants from superfoods like chia seeds, hemp hearts, and berries. These ingredients can help reduce inflammation and improve overall health, which can help prevent cancer. Plus, it's a delicious way to start your day!

Avocado Toast with Greens

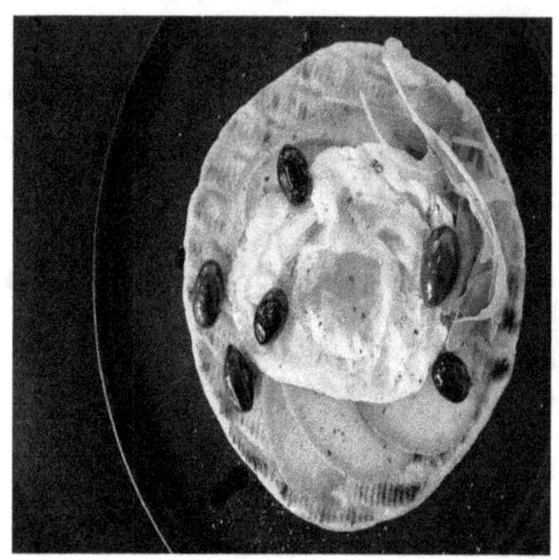

Prep time: 10 minutes

Ingredients:

1 slice whole-grain bread (70 calories)
1/2 medium avocado, mashed (117 calories)
1/2 cup mixed greens (10 calories)
1/2 tbsp lemon juice (3 calories)
1/2 tbsp extra-virgin olive oil (60 calories)

Salt and black pepper, to taste
Total calories: 260

Instructions:

Toast the bread slice to your desired level of crispiness.

While the bread is toasting, mash half an avocado in a small bowl. Add lemon juice, olive oil, salt, and black pepper, and mix well.

Once the bread is toasted, spread the avocado mixture on top.

Top the avocado toast with mixed greens.

Season with additional salt and black pepper, if desired.

Enjoy your nutritious and delicious Avocado Toast with Greens cancer breakfast!

Eggs with Veggies and Whole Wheat Toast

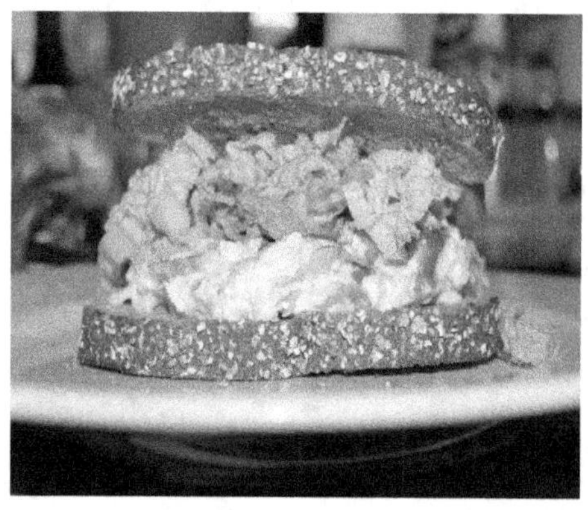

Prep time: 15 minutes

Ingredients:

2 large eggs
1/2 cup mixed veggies (such as bell peppers, onions, mushrooms, spinach)

1 slice whole wheat bread
1 tsp olive oil
Salt and pepper to taste
Calories count:

2 large eggs: 140 calories
1/2 cup mixed veggies: 25-50 calories
(depending on the veggies used)
1 slice whole wheat bread: 100-120 calories
(depending on the brand)
1 tsp olive oil: 40 calories (approx.)
Total: 305-350 calories

Instructions:

Heat a non-stick pan over medium heat and add 1 tsp of olive oil.

Add the mixed veggies to the pan and sauté for 5-7 minutes until they are tender and lightly browned.

In the meantime, toast the slice of whole wheat bread.

Crack the two eggs into the pan with the veggies and scramble them until fully cooked.

Season the eggs and veggies with salt and pepper to taste.

Serve the eggs and veggies on the slice of toasted whole wheat bread.

This recipe is high in protein and fiber, low in saturated fat, and provides a variety of essential vitamins and minerals from the veggies and whole wheat toast. It's a perfect healthy breakfast or brunch option that can help you feel satisfied and energized throughout the day!

Chapter 2: Appetizers and Snacks

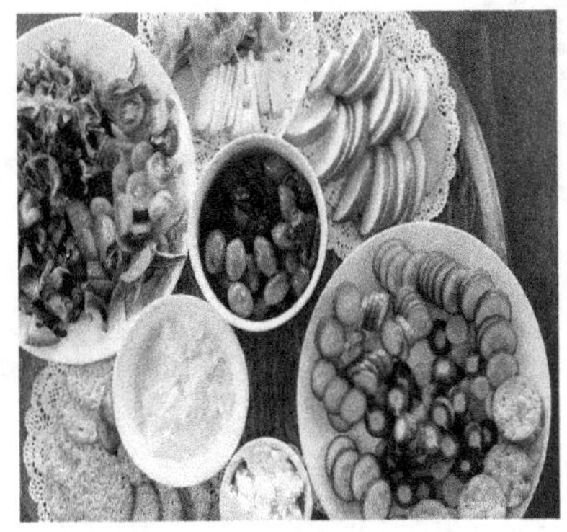

Guacamole with Fresh Veggies

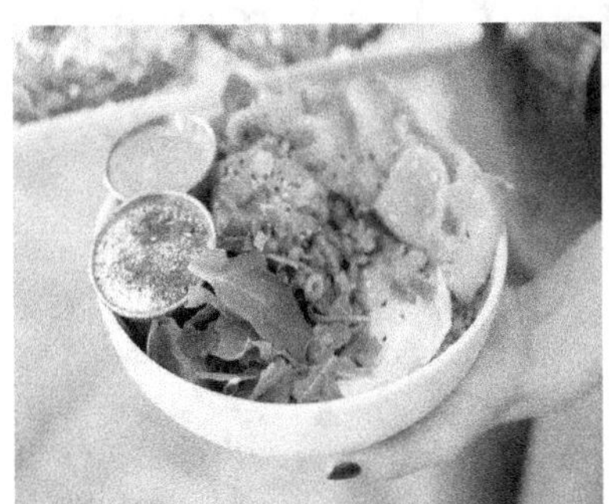

Ingredients:

2 ripe avocados
1 medium tomato, diced
1/4 cup diced red onion
1/4 cup chopped fresh cilantro
1 garlic clove, minced
1 jalapeno pepper, seeded and minced
Juice of 1 lime
Salt and pepper to taste
For serving:

Baby carrots
Cucumber slices
Red bell pepper strips
Preparation time: 10 minutes

Calories count (per serving): Approximately
165 calories

Instructions:

Cut the avocados in half and remove the pit. Scoop out the avocado flesh into a medium-sized bowl.

Add the diced tomato, red onion, cilantro, garlic, and jalapeno pepper to the bowl.
Squeeze the juice of one lime over the mixture and add salt and pepper to taste.
Mash the ingredients together with a fork until well combined, but still slightly chunky.

Serve the guacamole immediately with baby carrots, cucumber slices, and red bell pepper strips on the side for dipping.

This guacamole recipe is packed with cancer-fighting ingredients such as avocado, which is rich in antioxidants, and fresh veggies that are high in fiber and vitamins. Enjoy!

Cancer-Friendly Hummus Recipe.

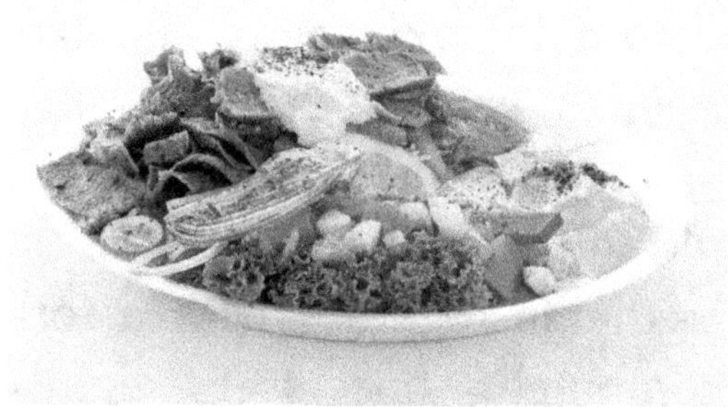

Ingredients:

1 can (15 oz) of chickpeas, drained and rinsed
2 cloves of garlic, minced
1/4 cup of tahini
1/4 cup of fresh lemon juice
2 tablespoons of extra-virgin olive oil
1/4 teaspoon of salt
1/4 teaspoon of ground cumin
1/4 teaspoon of paprika oo
2 whole wheat pita breads

Instructions:

In a food processor or blender, combine the chickpeas, garlic, tahini, lemon juice, olive oil, salt, cumin, and paprika. Process until smooth.
If the hummus is too thick, add a tablespoon of water at a time until the desired consistency is reached.
Cut the whole wheat pita breads into wedges and serve with the hummus.
Prep time: 10 minutes

Calories:

1 can of chickpeas: 285 calories
2 cloves of garlic: 9 calories
1/4 cup of tahini: 260 calories
1/4 cup of fresh lemon juice: 13 calories
2 tablespoons of extra-virgin olive oil: 238 calories
2 whole wheat pita breads: 320 calories
Total: 1,125 calories (for the entire recipe)

Roasted Chickpeas with Spices

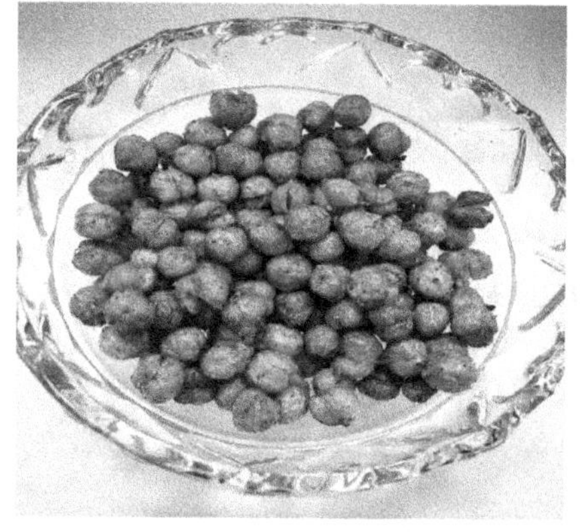

Prep Time: 10 minutes
Cook Time: 30 minutes
Total Time: 40 minutes
Servings: 4

Ingredients:
2 cans (15.5 oz each) chickpeas, drained and
rinsed

1 tablespoon olive oil
1 teaspoon ground cumin
1 teaspoon smoked paprika
1/2 teaspoon garlic powder
1/2 teaspoon onion powder
1/4 teaspoon cayenne pepper
Salt and black pepper, to taste
Fresh parsley, chopped (optional)

Instructions:

Preheat your oven to 400°F (200°C).
Drain and rinse the chickpeas, then pat them dry with a paper towel.

In a large mixing bowl, combine the chickpeas, olive oil, cumin, smoked paprika, garlic powder, onion powder, cayenne pepper, salt, and black pepper.

Mix well to coat the chickpeas evenly.
Transfer the seasoned chickpeas to a baking sheet lined with parchment paper or a silicone baking mat.

Roast the chickpeas in the oven for 25-30 minutes, or until they are crispy and golden brown. Shake the baking sheet halfway through the cooking time to ensure even browning.

Remove the roasted chickpeas from the oven and let them cool for a few minutes before serving. Garnish with chopped parsley, if desired.

Nutrition Information (per serving):

Calories: 191
Total Fat: 6g
Saturated Fat: 1g
Cholesterol: 0mg
Sodium: 289mg
Total Carbohydrates: 26g
Dietary Fiber: 7g
Sugars: 1g
Protein: 8g

Note: This recipe is a healthy and flavorful snack option for cancer patients as chickpeas are high in protein and fiber, which can help with digestion and promote feelings of fullness. The spices used in this recipe also provide anti-inflammatory and antioxidant benefits that can support overall health and well-being.

Veggie Chips and Salsa

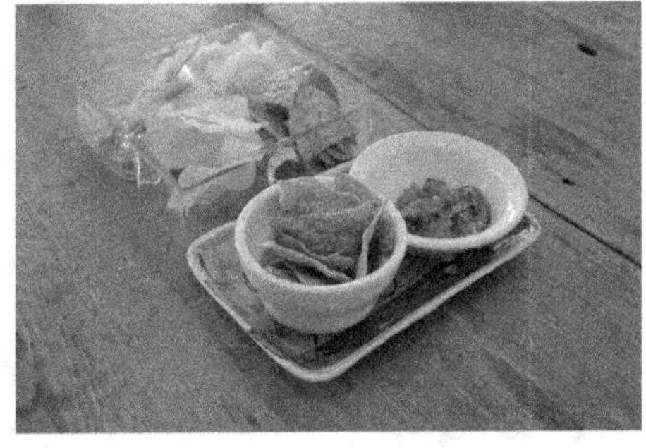

Ingredients for Veggie Chips:

1 large sweet potato
1 large beetroot
1 tablespoon olive oil
1/2 teaspoon sea salt

Ingredients for Salsa:

2 ripe tomatoes, diced
1/2 red onion, finely chopped
1/2 red bell pepper, finely chopped
1 jalapeño pepper, seeded and finely chopped
2 cloves garlic, minced
Juice of 1 lime
1/4 teaspoon sea salt
1/4 teaspoon black pepper
1/4 cup chopped fresh cilantro

Preparation:

Preheat the oven to 375°F (190°C). Line a large baking sheet with parchment paper.

Peel the sweet potato and beetroot, and slice them into thin rounds using a mandoline or sharp knife.

In a large bowl, toss the sweet potato and beetroot slices with olive oil and sea salt until evenly coated.

Arrange the slices in a single layer on the prepared baking sheet.

Bake for 20-25 minutes, flipping once halfway through, until the veggie chips are golden and crispy.

While the veggie chips are baking, prepare the salsa. In a medium bowl, combine the diced tomatoes, red onion, red bell pepper, jalapeño pepper, minced garlic, lime juice, sea salt, black pepper, and chopped cilantro. Mix well.

Serve the veggie chips warm with the salsa on the side for dipping.

Calories Count:

1 serving of Veggie Chips with Salsa (1/4 of the recipe) contains approximately 150 calories.
Each serving also provides a good source of dietary fiber, vitamins, and minerals from the sweet potato, beetroot, and fresh vegetables in the salsa.

Energy Bites with Nuts and Dried Fruit

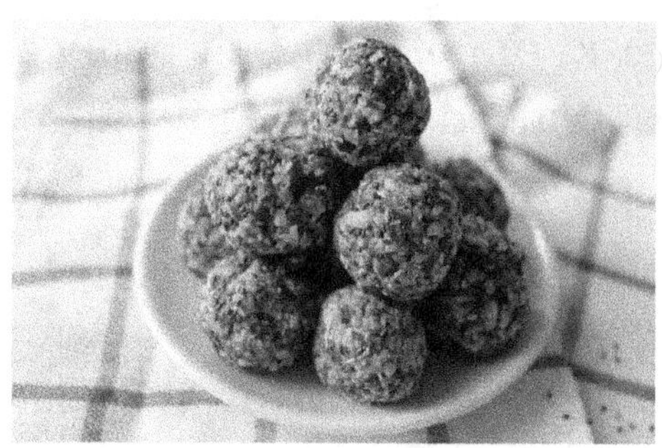

Ingredients:

1 cup of rolled oats
1/2 cup of unsweetened shredded coconut
1/2 cup of chopped nuts (such as almonds, walnuts, or pecans)
1/2 cup of chopped dried fruit (such as dates, apricots, or figs)
1/4 cup of ground flaxseed
1/4 cup of honey or maple syrup
1/4 cup of almond butter or peanut butter
1 tsp of vanilla extract
1/4 tsp of sea salt
Instructions:

In a large bowl, mix together the rolled oats, shredded coconut, chopped nuts, chopped dried fruit, and ground flaxseed.

In a separate bowl, mix together the honey or maple syrup, almond butter or peanut butter, vanilla extract, and sea salt.

Pour the wet ingredients over the dry ingredients and mix until well combined.

Use your hands to form the mixture into small balls, about 1 inch in diameter.

Place the balls on a baking sheet lined with parchment paper and refrigerate for at least 30 minutes to set.

Once set, the energy bites can be stored in an airtight container in the refrigerator for up to 1 week.

Prep time: Approximately 15 minutes

Calories per serving (1 energy bite): Approximately 100-120 calories, depending on the size and ingredients used.

Chapter 3: Salads and Dressings

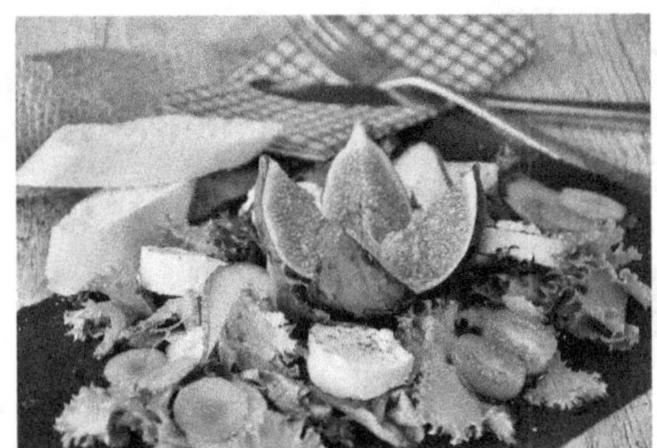

Greek Salad with Grilled Chicken

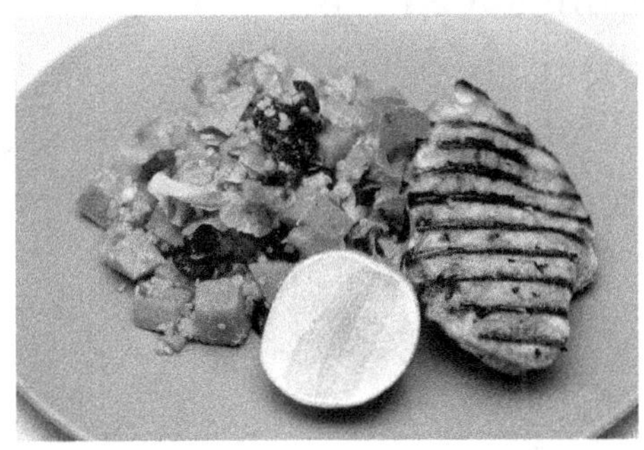

Prep time: 20 minutes
Cook time: 15 minutes
Total time: 35 minutes
Serves: 4

Ingredients:

2 boneless, skinless chicken breasts
2 teaspoons dried oregano
1 teaspoon garlic powder
1/2 teaspoon salt
1/4 teaspoon black pepper
1/4 cup olive oil
3 tablespoons lemon juice
1 tablespoon red wine vinegar
1 medium head of lettuce, chopped
1 medium cucumber, diced
1 medium red onion, sliced
1 large tomato, diced
1/2 cup crumbled feta cheese
1/4 cup Kalamata olives, pitted
1/4 cup chopped fresh parsley

Instructions:

Preheat the grill to medium-high heat.
In a small bowl, combine oregano, garlic powder, salt, pepper, olive oil, lemon juice, and red wine vinegar to make the marinade.

Place chicken breasts in a large resealable bag and pour the marinade over the chicken. Seal the bag and massage the marinade into the chicken until well coated. Allow the chicken to marinate in the fridge for 10-15 minutes.

Once the grill is hot, grill the chicken for about 6-8 minutes per side, or until the internal temperature reaches 165°F (75°C). Remove from heat and let rest for 5 minutes before slicing.

While the chicken is grilling assemble the salad by mixing the lettuce, cucumber, red onion, and tomato in a large bowl.

Top the salad with sliced grilled chicken, crumbled feta cheese, Kalamata olives, and chopped fresh parsley.

Serve the Greek salad with grilled chicken immediately and enjoy!

Nutrition Information (per serving):
Calories: 320
Total Fat: 21g
Saturated Fat: 6g
Cholesterol: 78mg
Sodium: 612mg
Total Carbohydrates: 9g
Dietary Fiber: 3g
Sugar: 5g
Protein: 26g

Note: Nutrition information is an estimate and may vary depending on specific ingredients used.

Rainbow Salad with Quinoa

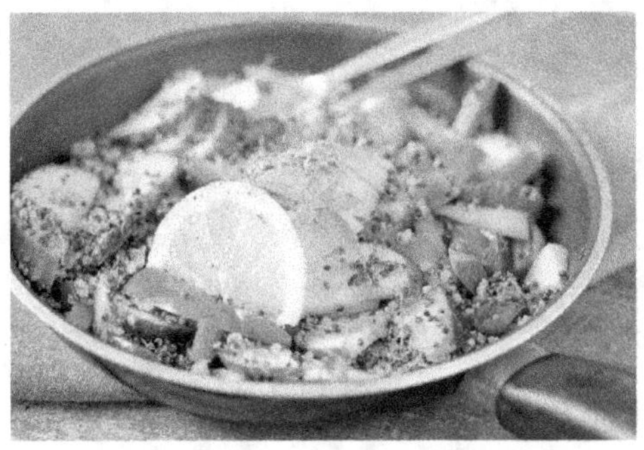

Prep time: 15 minutes

Ingredients:

1 cup cooked quinoa
2 cups baby spinach leaves
1 medium sized carrot, grated
1 medium sized beetroot, grated
1/2 red bell pepper, chopped
1/2 yellow bell pepper, chopped
1/2 cup cherry tomatoes, halved
1/4 cup chopped fresh parsley

1/4 cup chopped fresh mint
1/4 cup chopped fresh basil
2 tablespoons extra-virgin olive oil
1 tablespoon freshly squeezed lemon juice
Salt and pepper to taste

Instructions:

Cook the quinoa according to package instructions, set aside to cool.
In a large mixing bowl, combine the cooked quinoa, baby spinach leaves, grated carrot and beetroot, chopped bell peppers, cherry tomatoes, parsley, mint, and basil.

In a separate small bowl, whisk together the olive oil, lemon juice, salt, and pepper.
Pour the dressing over the salad and toss to combine.
Serve chilled.

Calories per serving: Approximately 250 calories per serving (recipe serves 4)

This recipe is a great option for those looking for a healthy and nutritious meal. Quinoa is a great source of plant-based protein, while the vegetables provide an array of vitamins and minerals. Plus, the colorful ingredients make for a visually appealing dish.

Spinach Salad with Berries and Nuts

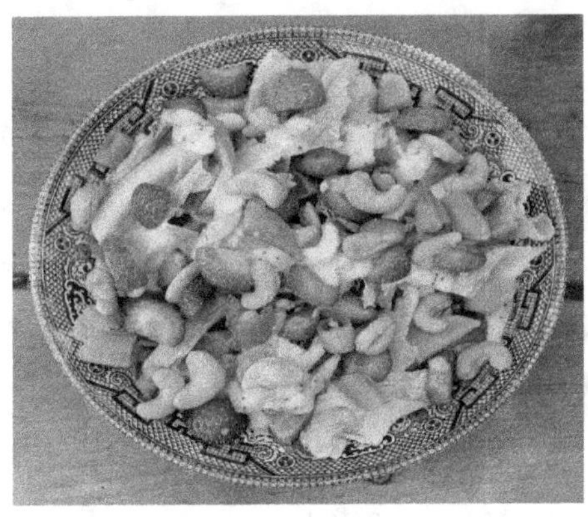

Prep time: 10 minutes

Ingredients:
4 cups baby spinach leaves
1 cup mixed berries (blueberries, strawberries, raspberries, blackberries)
1/4 cup chopped walnuts
1/4 cup crumbled feta cheese
1/4 cup balsamic vinaigrette dressing
Salt and pepper to taste

Instructions:
Rinse the spinach leaves thoroughly and pat dry with a paper towel. Place the spinach leaves in a large salad bowl.

Rinse the mixed berries and add them to the salad bowl.

Sprinkle the chopped walnuts and crumbled feta cheese over the top of the salad.
Drizzle the balsamic vinaigrette dressing over the top of the salad and toss until all the ingredients are evenly coated.

Season with salt and pepper to taste.

Calories: Approximately 200 calories per serving (serves 4)

Caesar Salad with Whole Grain Croutons

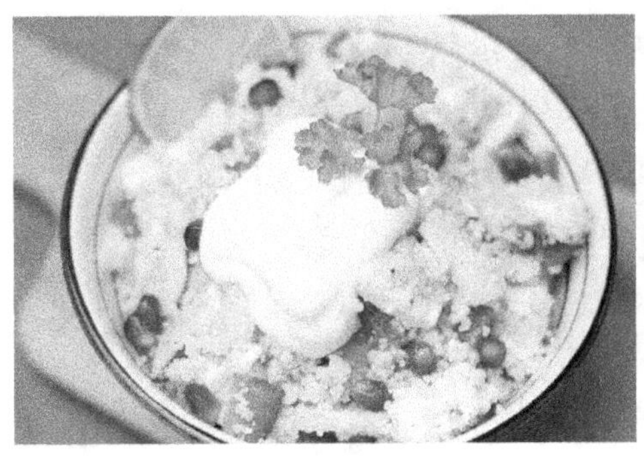

Prep Time: 20 minutes

Ingredients:

For the Salad:

1 head of romaine lettuce, chopped
1/2 cup cherry tomatoes, halved
1/4 cup red onion, thinly sliced
1/4 cup shredded parmesan cheese
For the Dressing:

1/4 cup plain Greek yogurt
1/4 cup olive oil
2 tablespoons fresh lemon juice
1 tablespoon Dijon mustard
2 cloves garlic, minced
1 teaspoon anchovy paste (optional)
Salt and black pepper, to taste
For the Whole Grain Croutons:

4 slices whole grain bread, cut into small cubes
1 tablespoon olive oil
1/4 teaspoon garlic powder
Salt and black pepper, to taste

Directions:

Preheat the oven to 375°F (190°C).

To make the whole grain croutons, toss the bread cubes with olive oil, garlic powder, salt, and black pepper in a bowl until evenly coated. Spread them in a single layer on a baking sheet and bake for 10-15 minutes, or until crispy and golden brown. Set aside to cool.

To make the dressing, whisk together the Greek yogurt, olive oil, lemon juice, Dijon mustard, garlic, anchovy paste (if using), salt, and black pepper in a small bowl until smooth and creamy.

To assemble the salad, place the chopped romaine lettuce in a large bowl. Add the cherry tomatoes, red onion, and shredded parmesan cheese. Drizzle the dressing over the salad and toss well to coat.

Top the salad with the whole grain croutons and serve immediately.

Calories: Approximately 260 calories per serving (recipe yields 4 servings)

Balsamic Vinaigrette Dressing

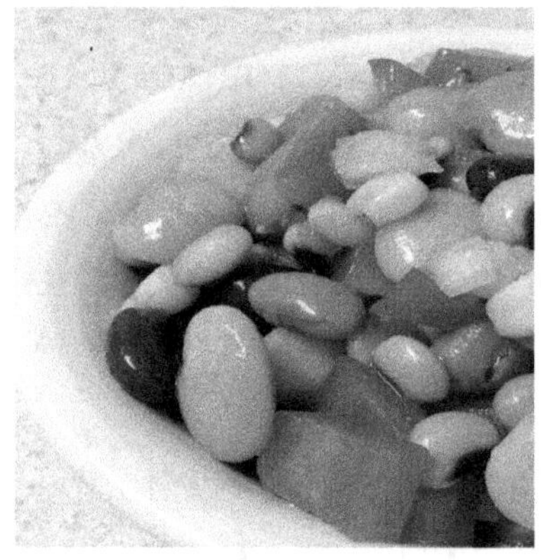

Prep Time: 5 minutes

Ingredients:

1/4 cup balsamic vinegar
1/4 cup extra-virgin olive oil

1 tablespoon Dijon mustard
1 tablespoon honey
1 small garlic clove, minced
Salt and freshly ground black pepper to taste

Preparation:

In a small bowl, whisk together the balsamic vinegar, Dijon mustard, honey, minced garlic, salt, and black pepper.
Slowly pour in the olive oil while whisking continuously until the mixture is emulsified.
Taste and adjust seasoning as needed.
Pour the dressing over your favorite salad and toss to combine.

Calories Count: This recipe makes approximately 4 servings, with each serving containing around 120 calories. Please note that this calorie count may vary depending on the exact brands and quantities of ingredients used.

Lemon-Herb Dressing

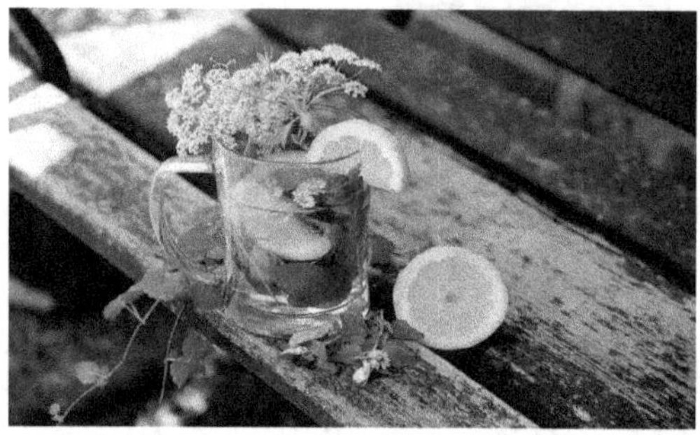

Prep Time: 10 minutes

Ingredients:

1/4 cup fresh lemon juice
2 tablespoons honey
1 tablespoon Dijon mustard
1 garlic clove, minced
1/4 teaspoon salt
1/4 teaspoon black pepper
1/2 cup extra-virgin olive oil
2 tablespoons chopped fresh herbs (such as parsley, thyme, and basil)

Instructions:

In a small bowl, whisk together the lemon juice, honey, Dijon mustard, garlic, salt, and black pepper until well combined.
Slowly pour in the olive oil while whisking constantly to emulsify the dressing.
Stir in the chopped herbs.

Taste and adjust seasoning as needed.
Use immediately or store in an airtight container in the refrigerator for up to 1 week.

Calories: This recipe makes approximately 8 servings, and each serving is about 120 calories.

This dressing is perfect for salads, roasted vegetables, grilled meats, and more! It's also rich in antioxidants and anti-inflammatory compounds, which can help reduce the risk of cancer and other chronic diseases. Enjoy!

Chapter 4: Soups and Stews

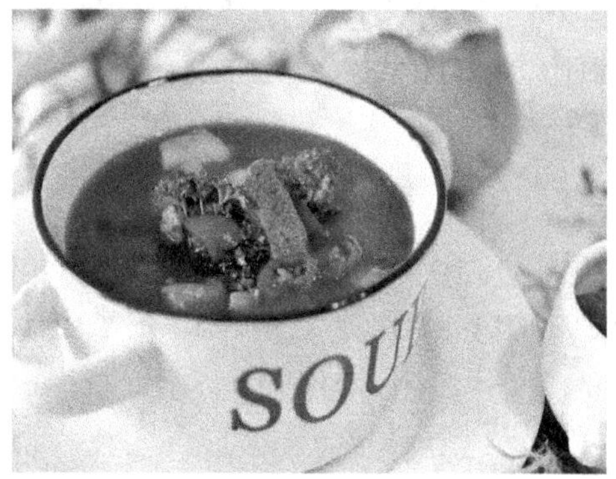

Vegetable Soup with Lentils

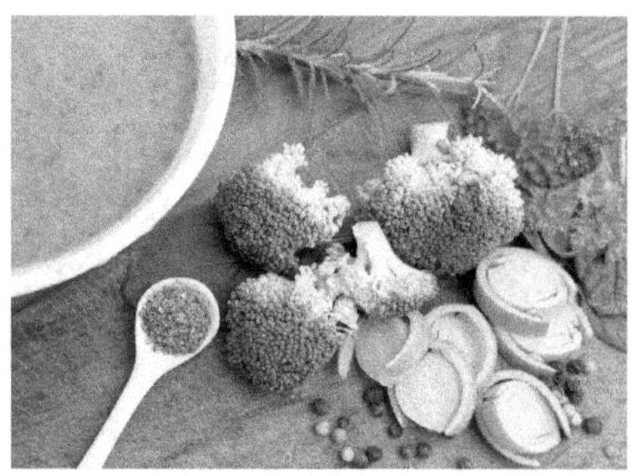

Prep time: 20 minutes
Cook time: 40 minutes
Total time: 60 minutes
Servings: 6

Ingredients:

1 tablespoon olive oil
1 large onion, diced
4 garlic cloves, minced
3 carrots, peeled and diced
3 celery stalks, diced
1 red bell pepper, diced
1 yellow bell pepper, diced
2 zucchinis, diced
1 can (14 oz) diced tomatoes
1 cup brown lentils, rinsed and drained
6 cups vegetable broth
1 teaspoon dried thyme
1 teaspoon dried oregano
Salt and pepper, to taste
Fresh parsley, chopped, for garnish

Instructions:

In a large pot, heat the olive oil over medium heat. Add the onion and garlic and sauté until the onion is translucent.

Add the carrots, celery, red and yellow bell peppers, and zucchini. Sauté for a few minutes until the vegetables start to soften.

Add the diced tomatoes, lentils, vegetable broth, thyme, and oregano. Stir to combine and bring to a boil.

Reduce the heat to low, cover the pot, and simmer for about 30 minutes, or until the lentils are tender.

Season with salt and pepper, to taste.

Ladle the soup into bowls and garnish with fresh parsley.

Nutrition information per serving (1/6 of recipe):
Calories: 200
Total fat: 3g
Saturated fat: 0g
Cholesterol: 0mg
Sodium: 480mg
Total carbohydrate: 35g
Dietary fiber: 12g
Sugars: 10g
Protein: 11g

Note: The calorie count is approximate and may vary depending on the exact ingredients used.

Chicken Noodle Soup with Veggies

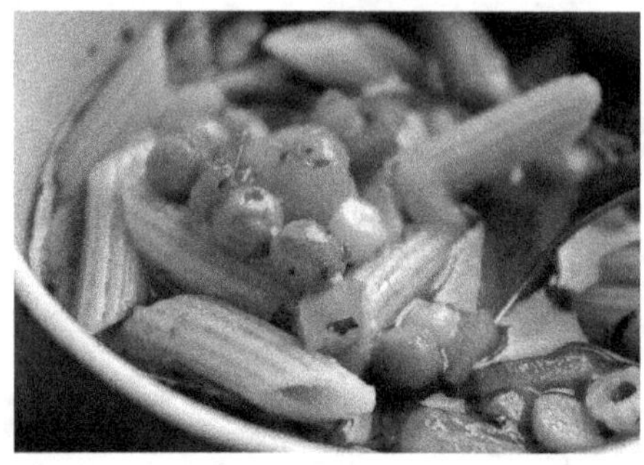

Prep time: 15 minutes

Ingredients:

1 tablespoon olive oil
1 onion, chopped
2 carrots, peeled and sliced
2 celery stalks, sliced
2 cloves garlic, minced
1 teaspoon dried thyme
8 cups low-sodium chicken broth
2 cups cooked shredded chicken breast
2 cups uncooked egg noodles
2 cups chopped kale
Salt and pepper, to taste

Instructions:

In a large pot, heat the olive oil over medium heat. Add the onion, carrots, and celery and sauté until tender, about 5 minutes.

Add the garlic and thyme and sauté for another minute.

Add the chicken broth and bring to a boil. Reduce the heat and simmer for 10 minutes.

Add the cooked shredded chicken and uncooked egg noodles and simmer for another 10 minutes or until the noodles are cooked.

Add the chopped kale and cook for an additional 2-3 minutes, or until the kale is wilted.

Season with salt and pepper to taste.

Serve hot.

Calories per serving (6 servings): 238 calories

Tomato Soup with Whole Grain Crackers

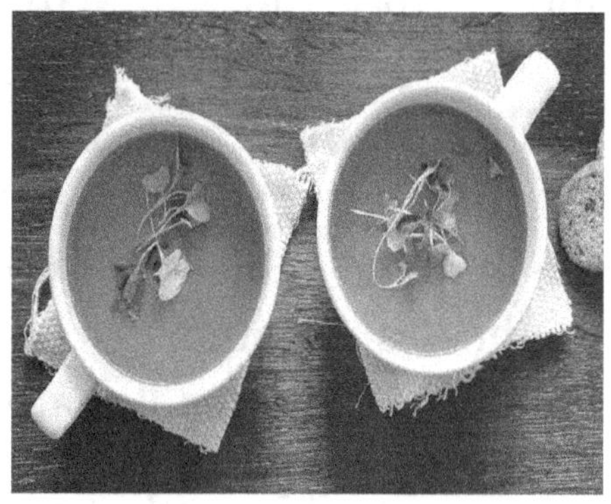

Ingredients:

2 tablespoons olive oil
1 large onion, chopped
4 cloves garlic, minced
2 cans (28 oz each) crushed tomatoes
2 cups chicken or vegetable broth
1 teaspoon dried basil
1 teaspoon dried oregano

1 teaspoon dried thyme
1/4 teaspoon red pepper flakes
1/2 teaspoon salt
1/4 teaspoon black pepper
1/2 cup plain Greek yogurt
2 tablespoons chopped fresh parsley
Whole grain crackers for serving
Preparation Time: 30 minutes

Calories count: 300 per serving

Instructions:

In a large pot, heat the olive oil over medium heat. Add the onion and garlic and sauté until softened, about 5 minutes.

Add the crushed tomatoes, broth, basil, oregano, thyme, red pepper flakes, salt, and black pepper. Stir to combine and bring to a simmer.

Cover and cook over low heat for 15 minutes.

Remove from heat and let cool slightly.

Puree the soup in batches in a blender or with an immersion blender until smooth.

Return the pureed soup to the pot and stir in the Greek yogurt.

Reheat over low heat until warmed through.

Serve hot with whole grain crackers on the side.

Beef Stew with Root Vegetables

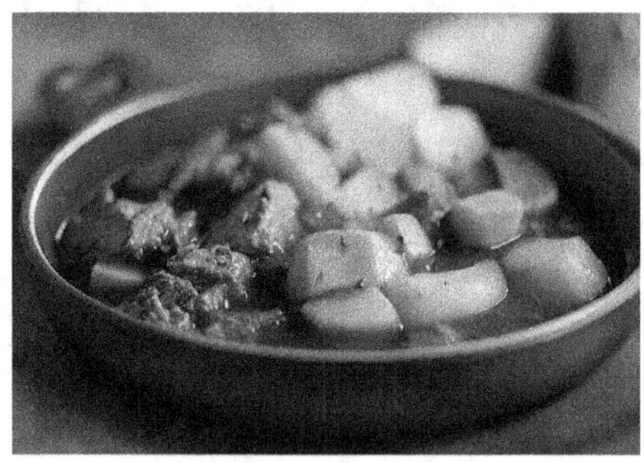

Prep time: 30 minutes
Cook time: 2 hours
Total time: 2 hours 30 minutes

Ingredients:

1.5 pounds beef stew meat, cut into 1-inch cubes
2 tablespoons olive oil
1 onion, chopped
2 cloves garlic, minced
3 carrots, peeled and sliced
3 parsnips, peeled and sliced
2 turnips, peeled and chopped
2 potatoes, peeled and chopped
4 cups beef broth
1 cup red wine
1 tablespoon tomato paste
2 bay leaves
1 teaspoon dried thyme
Salt and pepper, to taste

Instructions:

Heat the olive oil in a large pot or Dutch oven over medium-high heat.
Add the beef and cook until browned on all sides, about 5-7 minutes.
Add the onion and garlic and cook until softened, about 3-5 minutes.
Add the carrots, parsnips, turnips, and potatoes, and cook for another 5-7 minutes.

Add the beef broth, red wine, tomato paste, bay leaves, thyme, salt, and pepper to the pot.

Bring the stew to a boil, then reduce the heat to low and simmer for 2 hours, or until the beef is tender and the vegetables are cooked through.
Remove the bay leaves before serving.

Calories:
The calorie count for this recipe depends on the specific ingredients and serving size. However, based on an estimate, each

serving of this beef stew (assuming 6 servings in total) is approximately 400-500 calories

Lentil Stew with Spinach

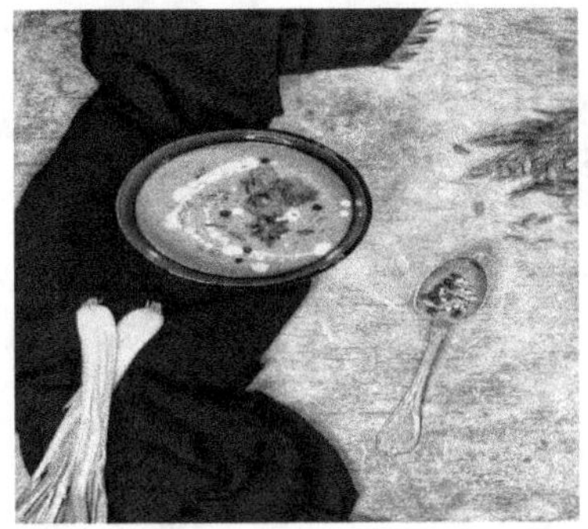

Prep time: 15 minutes
Cook time: 45 minutes
Total time: 1 hour

Ingredients:

1 cup dry lentils, rinsed and drained
1 tbsp olive oil
1 onion, chopped
2 cloves garlic, minced

2 celery stalks, chopped
2 carrots, chopped
1 tsp ground cumin
1 tsp ground coriander
1/2 tsp smoked paprika
1/2 tsp dried thyme
1 bay leaf
4 cups low-sodium vegetable broth
2 cups packed fresh spinach leaves, washed and chopped
Salt and pepper to taste
Instructions:

In a large pot, heat olive oil over medium heat. Add onions and garlic, and sauté until onions are translucent.

Add celery and carrots, and cook for 5 minutes, stirring occasionally.

Add cumin, coriander, smoked paprika, thyme, bay leaf, and lentils. Stir well to coat the lentils with the spices.

Add vegetable broth and bring to a boil. Reduce heat to low and let simmer for 30-40 minutes, or until lentils are tender.

Add spinach and cook for 5 more minutes, until spinach is wilted.

Remove bay leaf and season with salt and pepper to taste.

Serve hot, garnished with fresh herbs if desired.

Calories per serving: 234 calories (based on 6 servings)

Chapter 5: Main Dishes

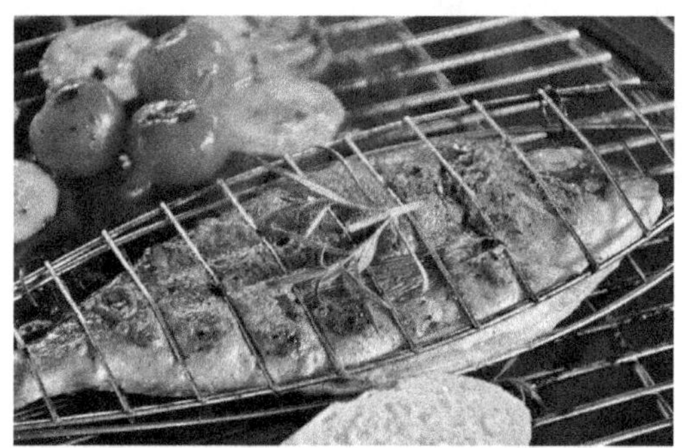

Grilled Salmon with Brown Rice and Steamed Veggies

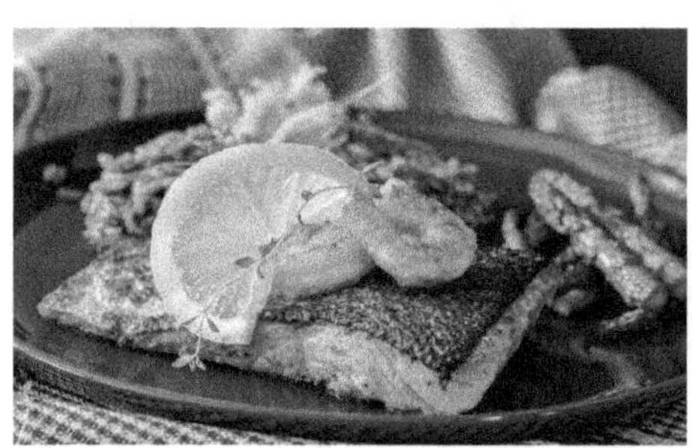

Prep time: 10 minutes
Cook time: 15 minutes
Total time: 25 minutes

Ingredients:

4 salmon filets (4-6 ounces each)
1 tbsp olive oil
2 tbsp soy sauce
1 tbsp honey
1 clove garlic, minced
1 tbsp fresh ginger, minced
2 cups cooked brown rice
4 cups mixed vegetables (such as broccoli, carrots, and zucchini), chopped
Salt and pepper to taste
Instructions:

Preheat grill to medium-high heat.

In a small bowl, whisk together olive oil, soy sauce, honey, garlic, and ginger.

Season salmon filets with salt and pepper, then brush both sides with the marinade.

Grill salmon for 4-6 minutes per side, or until cooked through.

While the salmon is grilling, steam mixed vegetables until tender, about 5-7 minutes.

Serve grilled salmon with cooked brown rice and steamed veggies on the side.

Calories per serving: 450 calories (based on 4 servings)

Whole Wheat Pasta with Tomato Sauce and Grilled Chicken

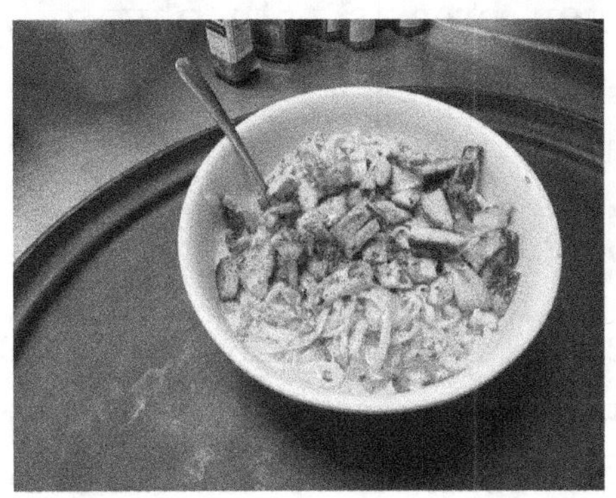

Ingredients:

8 oz. whole wheat pasta
2 cups of tomato sauce (homemade or store-bought, low-sodium if possible)
2 boneless, skinless chicken breasts
1 tablespoon olive oil
Salt and pepper to taste
Fresh basil (optional)

Instructions:

Cook the pasta according to the package directions, then drain and set aside.

Preheat your grill to medium-high heat.

Season the chicken breasts with olive oil, salt, and pepper.

Grill the chicken for about 6-7 minutes per side, or until the internal temperature reaches 165°F.

Let the chicken rest for a few minutes, then slice it into thin pieces.

In a medium saucepan, heat the tomato sauce over low heat until it's warm.

To serve, divide the pasta between four plates, top each serving with a generous amount of tomato sauce, and add sliced grilled chicken on top.

Garnish with fresh basil, if desired.

Prep time: 25 minutes

Calories per serving (serves 4): Approximately 400 calories.

Stir-Fry with Tofu and Mixed Veggies

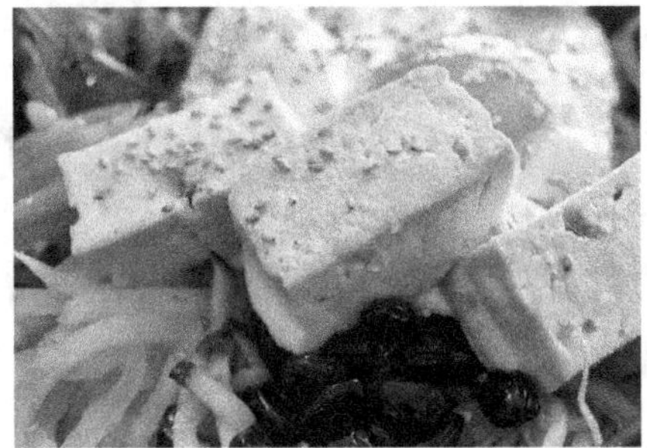

Prep Time: 20 minutes
Cook Time: 15 minutes
Total Time: 35 minutes
Servings: 4

Ingredients:

1 package of extra-firm tofu, drained and cut
into cubes
2 cups of mixed veggies (broccoli, carrots,
bell peppers, snap peas, etc.)
1 tablespoon of sesame oil
1 tablespoon of low-sodium soy sauce

1 teaspoon of minced garlic
1 teaspoon of grated ginger
Salt and pepper to taste
Brown rice, for serving

Instructions:

In a large skillet or wok, heat the sesame oil
over medium-high heat.
Add the garlic and ginger and cook for 30
seconds, stirring constantly.
Add the tofu and cook for 5-7 minutes, until
lightly browned and crispy on the outside.

Add the mixed veggies and soy sauce to the
skillet and stir-fry for 5-7 minutes, until the
veggies are tender but still crisp.
Season with salt and pepper to taste.
Serve the stir-fry over brown rice.

Nutrition Information:
Calories: 230 per serving
Total Fat: 10g
Saturated Fat: 1.5g

Cholesterol: 0mg
Sodium: 200mg
Total Carbohydrate: 18g
Dietary Fiber: 4g
Sugars: 4g
Protein: 20g

Turkey Chili with Beans and Whole Grain Bread

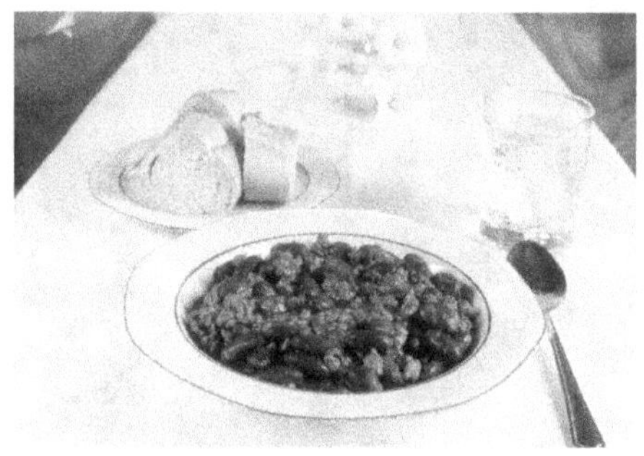

Preparation time: 30 minutes

Ingredients:

1 lb ground turkey
1 onion, diced
2 garlic cloves, minced
1 red bell pepper, diced
1 can of black beans, rinsed and drained
1 can of kidney beans, rinsed and drained
1 can of diced tomatoes

2 tablespoons chili powder
1 teaspoon ground cumin
1 teaspoon smoked paprika
1/2 teaspoon dried oregano
Salt and pepper to taste
Whole grain bread

Calories count: Approximately 400 calories per serving

Instructions:

Heat a large pot over medium heat. Add ground turkey and cook until browned, breaking up any large chunks with a spoon.

Add diced onion, minced garlic, and diced red bell pepper to the pot. Cook for 5-7 minutes, stirring occasionally, until the vegetables are softened.

Add the black beans, kidney beans, and diced tomatoes to the pot. Stir to combine.

Add chili powder, ground cumin, smoked paprika, dried oregano, salt, and pepper to the pot. Stir well to combine.

Bring the chili to a simmer and cook for 20-25 minutes, stirring occasionally, until the flavors have melded together and the chili has thickened.

Serve the chili hot with a slice of whole grain bread. Enjoy!

Baked Sweet Potato with Black Beans and Salsa

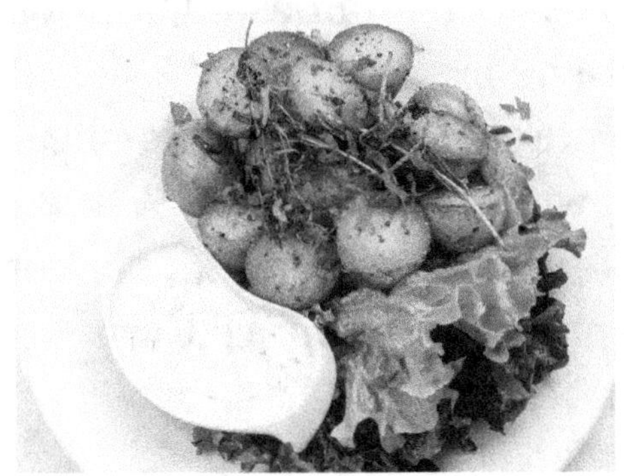

Prep time: 10 minutes
Cook time: 1 hour
Total time: 1 hour 10 minutes

Ingredients:

4 medium-sized sweet potatoes
1 can of black beans, drained and rinsed
1/2 cup of salsa
1/4 cup of chopped fresh cilantro
1 tablespoon of olive oil

Salt and pepper to taste

Instructions:

Preheat your oven to 400°F (200°C).
Wash and dry the sweet potatoes, then prick them all over with a fork.
Place the sweet potatoes on a baking sheet and drizzle them with olive oil.
Bake for 45 to 60 minutes or until the sweet potatoes are tender when pierced with a fork.

While the sweet potatoes are baking, prepare the black bean salsa. In a bowl, combine the black beans, salsa, and cilantro. Mix well.

Once the sweet potatoes are done, remove them from the oven and let them cool for a few minutes.
Slice the sweet potatoes lengthwise and gently fluff the flesh with a fork.

Spoon the black bean salsa over the sweet potatoes and season with salt and pepper to taste.
Serve immediately.

Calories count:

1 medium-sized sweet potato: approximately 100-130 calories
1/2 cup of black beans: approximately 110-120 calories
1/2 cup of salsa: approximately 30-50 calories
1/4 cup of chopped fresh cilantro: approximately 1-2 calories
1 tablespoon of olive oil: approximately 120 calories
Total calories count per serving: approximately 360-420 calories

Chapter 6: Desserts

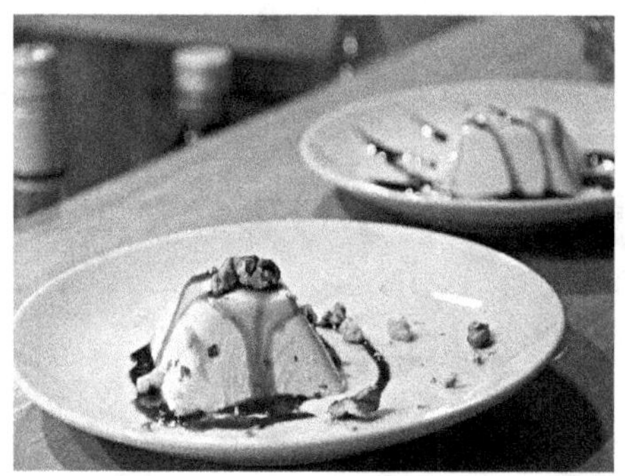

Fruit Salad with Yogurt and Granola

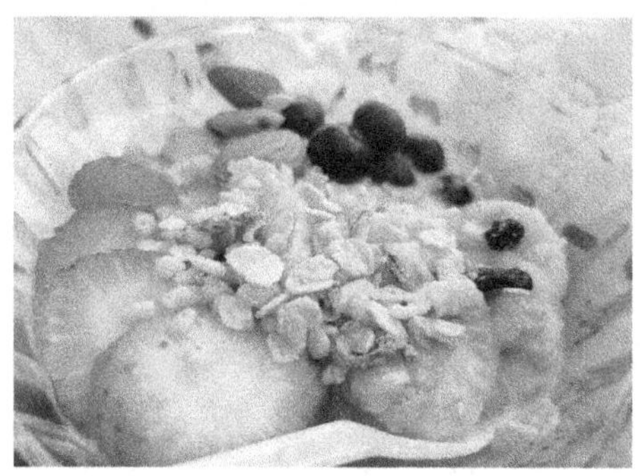

Prep time: 10 minutes
Serves: 4

Ingredients:

2 cups mixed berries (such as strawberries, blueberries, raspberries, and blackberries)
2 cups chopped fresh fruit (such as peaches, kiwi, pineapple, and mango)
1 cup plain Greek yogurt
2 tablespoons honey
1 teaspoon vanilla extract
1 cup granola
Fresh mint leaves (optional)
Instructions:

Wash and chop the fruits into bite-sized pieces and mix them together in a large bowl.

In a separate bowl, whisk together the Greek yogurt, honey, and vanilla extract until smooth.

Pour the yogurt mixture over the fruit and stir until well coated.

Sprinkle the granola over the top of the fruit and yogurt mixture.

Garnish with fresh mint leaves, if desired.

Chill in the refrigerator for 10-15 minutes before serving.

Nutrition information (per serving):
Calories: 292
Protein: 12g
Carbohydrates: 55g
Fat: 5g
Fiber: 7g

Chocolate Avocado Pudding

Prep time: 10 minutes

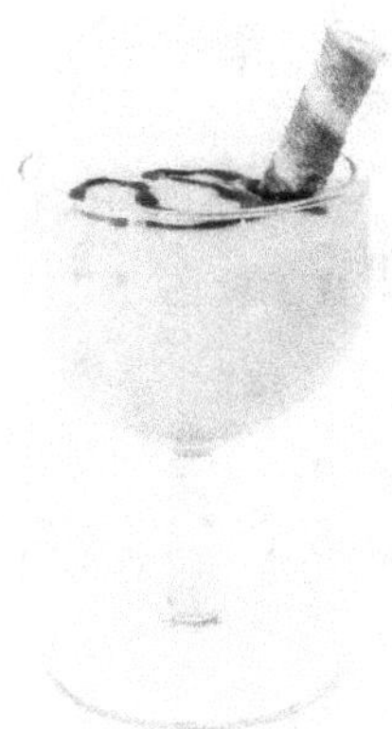

Ingredients:

2 ripe avocados
1/2 cup unsweetened cocoa powder
1/2 cup honey
1/2 cup almond milk
1 teaspoon vanilla extract
1/4 teaspoon salt
Instructions:

Cut the avocados in half, remove the pits, and scoop the flesh into a blender or food processor.

Add the cocoa powder, honey, almond milk, vanilla extract, and salt to the blender or food processor.

Blend or process until the ingredients are well combined and the pudding is smooth and creamy.

Taste the pudding and adjust the sweetness or cocoa powder to your liking.

Divide the pudding among four small bowls or ramekins and chill in the refrigerator for at least 30 minutes before serving.

Calories count: Approximately 250 calories per serving.

Banana-Oat Cookies with Raisins

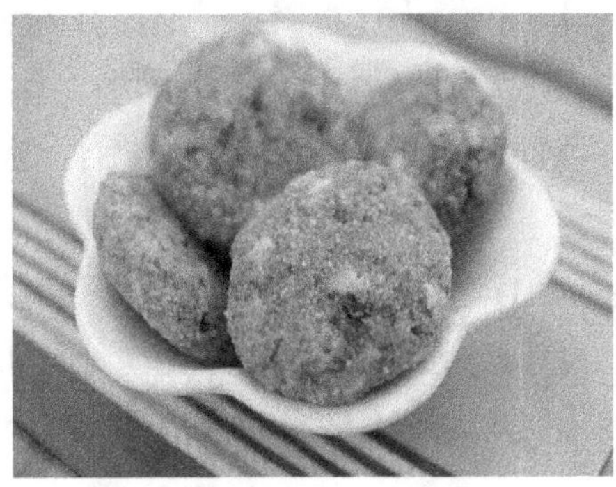

Prep Time: 10 minutes

Ingredients:

2 ripe bananas, mashed
1 cup rolled oats
1/2 cup raisins
1 teaspoon cinnamon
1/4 teaspoon nutmeg
1/4 teaspoon salt

Instructions:

Preheat the oven to 350°F (180°C) and line a baking sheet with parchment paper.

In a mixing bowl, combine the mashed bananas, rolled oats, raisins, cinnamon, nutmeg, and salt. Mix well until everything is evenly combined.

Using a cookie scoop or spoon, scoop the dough onto the prepared baking sheet and flatten each cookie slightly with your fingers.

Bake for 15-20 minutes, or until the edges are golden brown.

Allow the cookies to cool on the baking sheet for a few minutes before transferring them to a wire rack to cool completely.

Store the cookies in an airtight container at room temperature for up to 3 days, or freeze for longer storage.

Calories: Each cookie has approximately 85 calories.

Berry Crisp with Whole Grain Topping

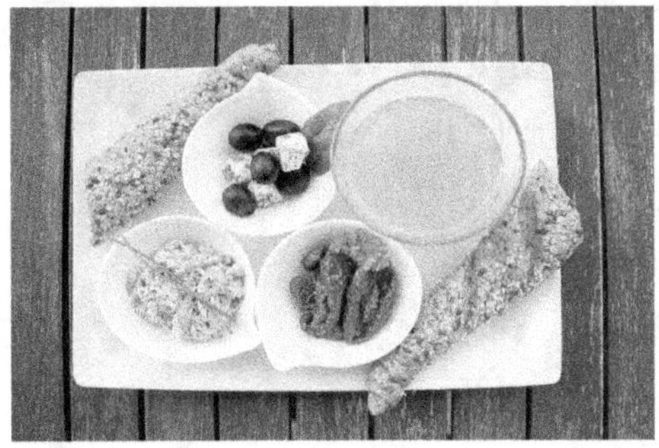

serves 6-8 people.
Prep time: 15 minutes

Ingredients:

For the Filling:

4 cups of mixed berries (such as strawberries, blueberries, raspberries, and blackberries)

2 tablespoons of honey
1 tablespoon of cornstarch
1 tablespoon of lemon juice

For the Topping:

1 cup of rolled oats
1/2 cup of whole wheat flour
1/2 cup of chopped almonds
1/4 cup of coconut oil (melted)
1/4 cup of honey
1 teaspoon of cinnamon
1/4 teaspoon of salt

Directions:

Preheat your oven to 375°F (190°C).
Rinse the mixed berries in cold water and drain them.

In a large mixing bowl, combine the berries, honey, cornstarch, and lemon juice. Mix well.

Spread the berry mixture evenly in a 9-inch baking dish.

In a separate mixing bowl, combine the rolled oats, whole wheat flour, chopped almonds, coconut oil, honey, cinnamon, and salt. Mix well.

Sprinkle the topping evenly over the berry mixture.

Bake for 30-35 minutes, or until the topping is golden brown and the berries are bubbly. Let the Berry Crisp cool for 5-10 minutes before serving.

Calories per serving (based on 8 servings): 254 calories

Pumpkin Pie with Whole Wheat Crust

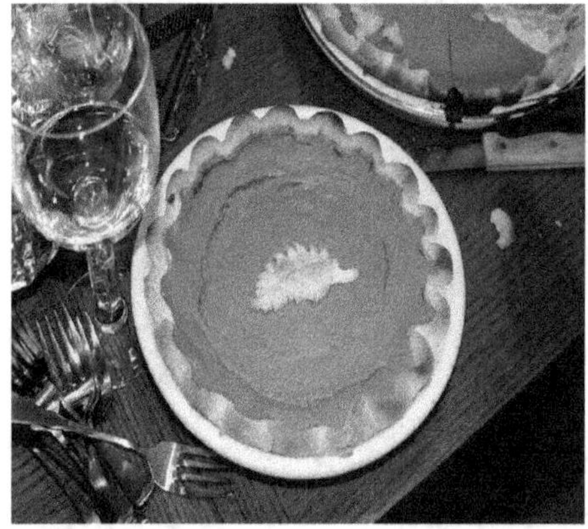

Prep time:15 minutes for the crust
10 minutes for the filling.
Baking time: 45 to 50 minutes.
Total time: 1 hour and 20 minutes.

Ingredients for Crust:

1 1/2 cups whole wheat flour
1/2 tsp salt

1/3 cup vegetable oil
3-4 tbsp cold water

Ingredients for Filling:

1 15-ounce can pumpkin puree
1/2 cup brown sugar
2 large eggs
1 tsp ground cinnamon
1/2 tsp ground ginger
1/4 tsp ground nutmeg
1/4 tsp salt
1 1/4 cups low-fat milk

Directions:

Preheat your oven to 375°F.
In a medium bowl, mix together the whole wheat flour and salt. Add the vegetable oil and stir until the mixture resembles coarse crumbs. Add cold water one tablespoon at a time, mixing until the dough comes together.

Roll out the dough on a floured surface, and place it into a 9-inch pie dish. Trim any excess dough from the edges.

In a large bowl, whisk together the pumpkin puree, brown sugar, eggs, cinnamon, ginger, nutmeg, and salt. Gradually stir in the low-fat milk until fully combined.

Pour the pumpkin mixture into the prepared pie crust.

Bake the pie for 45 to 50 minutes, or until the filling is set and the crust is golden brown.

Allow the pie to cool completely before slicing and serving.

Calories count: The whole pie contains approximately 1,100 calories, with each slice (if the pie is divided into 8 slices) containing approximately 138 calories. Please note that these are estimates and may vary depending on the specific ingredients used.

Chapter 7 Bonus/ Conclusion

Tips for Meal Planning and Preparation
Resources for Cancer Patients and Caregivers

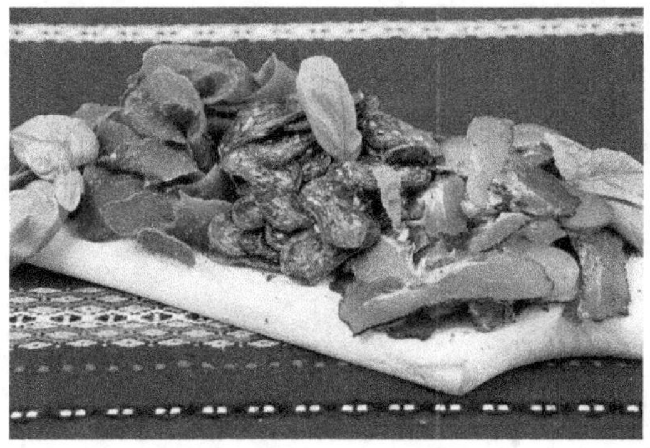

Tips for Meal Planning and Preparation:

Plan ahead: Take some time to plan your meals for the week. This will help you save time and money by allowing you to buy only what you need and avoid last-minute trips to the grocery store.

Choose healthy ingredients: Focus on fresh fruits, vegetables, whole grains, lean proteins, and healthy fats. These foods can help you maintain a healthy weight and reduce your risk of cancer and other diseases.

Keep it simple: You don't have to be a gourmet chef to prepare healthy meals. Simple meals, such as grilled chicken with roasted vegetables or a salad with grilled salmon, can be both healthy and delicious.

Batch cook: Prepare meals in advance and store them in the fridge or freezer for quick and easy meals during the week.

Get creative: Try new recipes and experiment with different ingredients to keep your meals interesting and flavorful.

Use healthy cooking methods: Choose cooking methods that preserve the nutrients in your food, such as steaming, grilling, or baking.

Don't skip meals: Eating regularly can help you maintain your energy levels and prevent overeating later in the day.

Resources for Cancer Patients and Caregivers:

American Cancer Society: The American Cancer Society provides information and resources for cancer patients and their families, including information about treatment options, managing side effects, and support groups.

CancerCare: CancerCare provides free professional support services for cancer patients and their caregivers, including counseling, support groups, and educational workshops.

National Cancer Institute: The National Cancer Institute provides information about cancer research, treatment options, and clinical trials.

Cancer Support Community: The Cancer Support Community offers support groups, educational programs, and resources for cancer patients and their families.

Livestrong Foundation: The Livestrong Foundation provides resources for cancer patients and survivors, including information about treatment options, financial assistance, and support groups.

Cancer.Net: Cancer.Net provides information and resources for cancer patients and their families, including information about treatment options, managing side effects, and coping with cancer.

Hospice Foundation of America: The Hospice Foundation of America provides information and resources for caregivers of terminally ill patients, including information about hospice care, grief support, and caregiver resources.